Skin Care

Herbs And Essential Oils for Natural Skin Care

Table of Contents

Introduction

You walk through the aisles, looking for something that's going to give you the moisture you want, without leaving your skin feeling heavy and greasy. You want something that's going to take care of dry skin, but you have always had trouble with acne, and you don't want to aggravate that in the process.

You walk through the aisles, looking for something that's going to get rid of the wrinkles that have formed on your face and the dark circles that have come under your eyes. You don't feel old enough to have these thin lines on your face, and you are ready to reverse the clock.

But when you see the products, all you see are things filled with chemicals. Things you don't want to put on your skin, and things you wish weren't there in place of things that actually work.

If only there was a way you could find natural remedies for your skin care needs. You have heard so many wonderful things about going the natural route, and you want to put it to the test, but all you see in the store are chemical products that cause countless side effects.

Well, you have come to the right place. With this book, you are going to learn how to use a variety of herbs and essential oils to take care of all your skin's needs.

From the dry skin to the blemishes to the wrinkles, herbs and essential oils have the power to remove them all, and leave you feeling fresh and clean.

This book is full of the recipes you need to enjoy skin like you once had. Tight, firm skin that is soft and smooth to the touch, without a single breakout, dark circle, or sun spot in sight.

These remedies are perfect for all, without any side effects or harmful chemicals that will cause more damage to your skin than good. You can feel great about putting these on your face and hands, and in no time at all you will see the benefits you have been hoping for.

I am going to show you the secret to total skin care, and by the time you reach the end of this book, you are going to say goodbye to the cosmetics you find on the shelves of the store for good.

There's no end to the ways you can experience all natural benefits with these

herbs and oils, and once you have tried them, you will never want to go back. Are you ready to dive into a world of all natural health that will give you the benefits you want?

Excellent.

Then let's get started.

Chapter 1 – A Word on Natural Remedies

In a world that is full of chemical cosmetics, it's a wonder natural remedies still exist. But they do, and with good reason. In spite of all the changes that have taken place in medicine and cosmetics these days, natural remedies are still an excellent option for those who want to do things without chemicals.

The remedies are still around because they work. They are going to give you the results you have been looking for, without costing you an arm and a leg, or causing you side effects that you would rather not experience.

Can I use these as often as I would like?

Yes, when it comes to natural remedies, you can use as much as you want because you don't have to worry about damaging your skin. You aren't ingesting them, you are mixing them with your favorite face soap and applying them to your skin, where they are going to provide tons of benefits without any harm.

Can I mix recipes to find what I want?

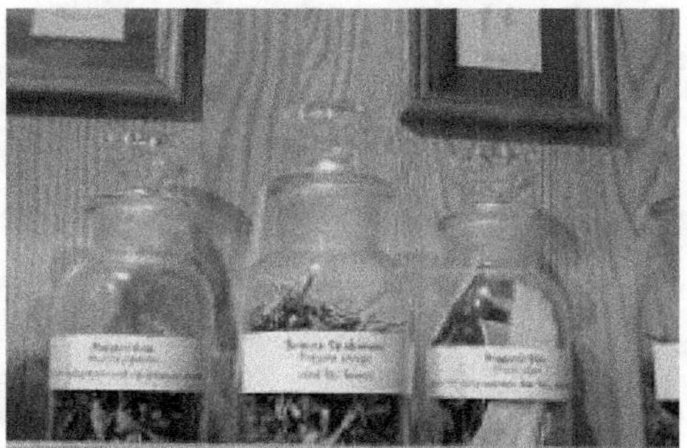

When you are making your own natural remedies, you can do whatever you want. If there is an ingredient you like from one recipe, and others you like from another, then go ahead and mix it up.

It's your skin, and all the oils and herbs in this book are excellent for any skin on your body, so have fun and see what blends you can create. One of the biggest benefits that comes with making your own remedies is that you have the freedom to do what you want, when you want.

Where do I get these oils and herbs?

With essential oils being so popular, you can find them in many local stores. These herbs can all be purchased in local health food stores or online, so you aren't going to have any issues finding what you are looking for.

You can buy them in bulk or buy a little at a time until you know what's right for you – either way, you are going to fall in love with the results.

So, if you are ready to break out of the modern way of doing things and start embracing remedies like others have done for centuries, we are ready to get into the recipes. As I said, try them all out for yourself, find your favorites, and use the recipes here as inspiration to make your own.

You can't go wrong with herbal remedies and essential oils, so give it all you got and let your creativity shine!

You deserve to be pampered.

Chapter 2 – Essential Oils For Life

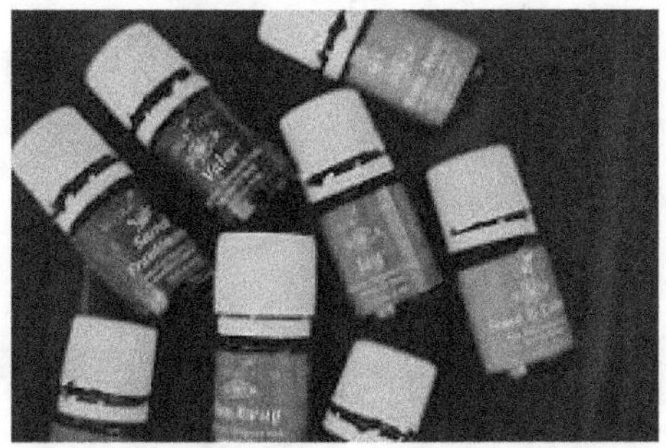

Forever 22
What you will need:

10 drops myrrh

10 drops vetiver oil

5 drops peppermint oil

1 tablespoon carrier oil of your choice (optional - this can be jojoba oil, sweet almond oil, or fractionated coconut oil)

Directions:

Combine the oils in a jar and shake well to combine. If you want to use only oils, combine with 1 tablespoon of a carrier oil, such as fractionated coconut oil or sweet almond oil.

You can also blend it with your favorite face soap or body wash and use it on your face, body, hands, and feet.

You can also combine with some water and diffuse it into the air, keeping the air in your house perfect for flawless and perfect skin.

The Blemish Banisher
What you will need:

10 drops frankincense oil

11 drops geranium oil

11 drops chamomile

1 tablespoon carrier oil of your choice (optional - this can be jojoba oil, sweet almond oil, or fractionated coconut oil)

Directions:

Combine the oils in a jar and shake well to combine. If you want to use only oils, combine with 1 tablespoon of a carrier oil, such as fractionated coconut oil or sweet almond oil.

You can also blend it with your favorite face soap or body wash and use it on your face, body, hands, and feet.

You can also combine with some water and diffuse it into the air, keeping the air in your house perfect for flawless and perfect skin.

Bright Eyes
What you will need:

10 drops rose oil

10 drops sandalwood oil

4 drops eucalyptus oil

1 tablespoon carrier oil of your choice (optional - this can be jojoba oil, sweet almond oil, or fractionated coconut oil)

Directions:

Combine the oils in a jar and shake well to combine. If you want to use only oils, combine with 1 tablespoon of a carrier oil, such as fractionated coconut oil or sweet almond oil.

You can also blend it with your favorite face soap or body wash and use it on your face, body, hands, and feet.

You can also combine with some water and diffuse it into the air, keeping the air in your house perfect for flawless and perfect skin.

Princess Skin

What you will need:

10 drops rosewood oil

5 drops basil oil

3 drops wintergreen oil

1 tablespoon carrier oil of your choice (optional - this can be jojoba oil, sweet almond oil, or fractionated coconut oil)

Directions:

Combine the oils in a jar and shake well to combine. If you want to use only oils, combine with 1 tablespoon of a carrier oil, such as fractionated coconut oil or sweet almond oil.

You can also blend it with your favorite face soap or body wash and use it on your face, body, hands, and feet.

You can also combine with some water and diffuse it into the air, keeping the air in your house perfect for flawless and perfect skin.

Sultry Smooth
What you will need:

10 drops vetiver oil

9 drops geranium oil

8 drops wintergreen oil

1 tablespoon carrier oil of your choice (optional - this can be jojoba oil, sweet almond oil, or fractionated coconut oil)

Directions:

Combine the oils in a jar and shake well to combine. If you want to use only oils, combine with 1 tablespoon of a carrier oil, such as fractionated coconut oil or sweet almond oil.

You can also blend it with your favorite face soap or body wash and use it on your face, body, hands, and feet.

You can also combine with some water and diffuse it into the air, keeping the air in your house perfect for flawless and perfect skin.

The Cure-All
What you will need:

10 drops lavender oil

10 drops ylang ylang oil

7 drops sandalwood oil

1 tablespoon carrier oil of your choice (optional - this can be jojoba oil, sweet almond oil, or fractionated coconut oil)

Directions:

Combine the oils in a jar and shake well to combine. If you want to use only oils, combine with 1 tablespoon of a carrier oil, such as fractionated coconut oil or sweet almond oil.

You can also blend it with your favorite face soap or body wash and use it on your face, body, hands, and feet.

You can also combine with some water and diffuse it into the air, keeping the air in your house perfect for flawless and perfect skin.

The Wrinkle Smoother
What you will need:

12 drops spearmint oil

11 drops cinnamon oil

3 drops tea tree oil

1 tablespoon carrier oil of your choice (optional - this can be jojoba oil, sweet almond oil, or fractionated coconut oil)

Directions:

Combine the oils in a jar and shake well to combine. If you want to use only oils, combine with 1 tablespoon of a carrier oil, such as fractionated coconut oil or sweet almond oil.

You can also blend it with your favorite face soap or body wash and use it on your face, body, hands, and feet.

You can also combine with some water and diffuse it into the air, keeping the air in your house perfect for flawless and perfect skin.

Mama's Secret

What you will need:

10 drops frankincense oil

8 drops sage oil

8 drops orange oil

1 tablespoon carrier oil of your choice (optional - this can be jojoba oil, sweet almond oil, or fractionated coconut oil)

Directions:

Combine the oils in a jar and shake well to combine. If you want to use only oils, combine with 1 tablespoon of a carrier oil, such as fractionated coconut oil or sweet almond oil.

You can also blend it with your favorite face soap or body wash and use it on your face, body, hands, and feet.

You can also combine with some water and diffuse it into the air, keeping the air in your house perfect for flawless and perfect skin.

The Age Defying Wizard

What you will need:

12 drops myrrh oil

11 drops lavender oil

5 drops chamomile oil

1 tablespoon carrier oil of your choice (optional - this can be jojoba oil, sweet almond oil, or fractionated coconut oil)

Directions:

Combine the oils in a jar and shake well to combine. If you want to use only oils, combine with 1 tablespoon of a carrier oil, such as fractionated coconut oil or sweet almond oil.

You can also blend it with your favorite face soap or body wash and use it on your face, body, hands, and feet.

You can also combine with some water and diffuse it into the air, keeping the air in your house perfect for flawless and perfect skin.

Winter Solstice

What you will need:

10 drops spearmint oil

10 drops peppermint oil

8 drops balsam fir oil

1 tablespoon carrier oil of your choice (optional - this can be jojoba oil, sweet almond oil, or fractionated coconut oil)

Directions:

Combine the oils in a jar and shake well to combine. If you want to use only oils, combine with 1 tablespoon of a carrier oil, such as fractionated coconut oil or sweet almond oil.

You can also blend it with your favorite face soap or body wash and use it on your face, body, hands, and feet.

You can also combine with some water and diffuse it into the air, keeping the air in your house perfect for flawless and perfect skin.

Rough Patch Savior

What you will need:

10 drops myrrh oil

10 drops geranium oil

10 drops rosewood oil

1 tablespoon carrier oil of your choice (optional - this can be jojoba oil, sweet almond oil, or fractionated coconut oil)

Directions:

Combine the oils in a jar and shake well to combine. If you want to use only oils, combine with 1 tablespoon of a carrier oil, such as fractionated coconut oil or sweet almond oil.

You can also blend it with your favorite face soap or body wash and use it on your face, body, hands, and feet.

You can also combine with some water and diffuse it into the air, keeping the air in your house perfect for flawless and perfect skin.

The Goddess

What you will need:

10 drops blood orange oil

10 drops lime oil

10 drops lemon oil

1 tablespoon carrier oil of your choice (optional - this can be jojoba oil, sweet almond oil, or fractionated coconut oil)

Directions:

Combine the oils in a jar and shake well to combine. If you want to use only oils, combine with 1 tablespoon of a carrier oil, such as fractionated coconut oil or sweet almond oil.

You can also blend it with your favorite face soap or body wash and use it on your face, body, hands, and feet.

You can also combine with some water and diffuse it into the air, keeping the air in your house perfect for flawless and perfect skin.

Penelope Blend
What you will need:

10 drops grapefruit oil

11 drops sweet orange oil

11 drops lemongrass oil

1 tablespoon carrier oil of your choice (optional - this can be jojoba oil, sweet almond oil, or fractionated coconut oil)

Directions:

Combine the oils in a jar and shake well to combine. If you want to use only oils, combine with 1 tablespoon of a carrier oil, such as fractionated coconut oil or sweet almond oil.

You can also blend it with your favorite face soap or body wash and use it on your face, body, hands, and feet.

You can also combine with some water and diffuse it into the air, keeping the air in your house perfect for flawless and perfect skin.

Happy Hands

What you will need:

10 drops sandalwood oil

11 drops cinnamon oil

10 drops patchouli oil

1 tablespoon carrier oil of your choice (optional - this can be jojoba oil, sweet almond oil, or fractionated coconut oil)

Directions:

Combine the oils in a jar and shake well to combine. If you want to use only oils, combine with 1 tablespoon of a carrier oil, such as fractionated coconut oil or sweet almond oil.

You can also blend it with your favorite face soap or body wash and use it on your face, body, hands, and feet.

You can also combine with some water and diffuse it into the air, keeping the air in your house perfect for flawless and perfect skin.

Head to Toe

What you will need:

10 drops vanilla oil

10 drops Douglas fir oil

11 drops pine oil

1 tablespoon carrier oil of your choice (optional - this can be jojoba oil, sweet almond oil, or fractionated coconut oil)

Directions:

Combine the oils in a jar and shake well to combine. If you want to use only oils, combine with 1 tablespoon of a carrier oil, such as fractionated coconut oil or sweet almond oil.

You can also blend it with your favorite face soap or body wash and use it on your face, body, hands, and feet.

You can also combine with some water and diffuse it into the air, keeping the air in your house perfect for flawless and perfect skin.

Chapter 3 – All About Those Herbs

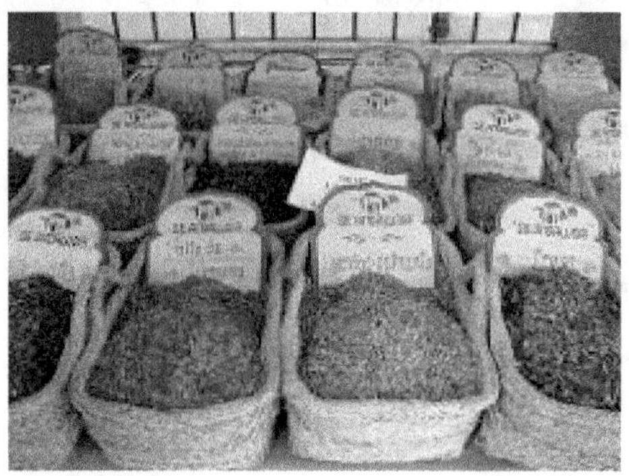

Super Tincture
What you will need:

1 teaspoon dried rose petals (dried)

1 teaspoon crushed rose hips

1 teaspoon dried chamomile leaves (dried)

Directions:

Crush the herbs and blend them with either your favorite moisturizing skin lotion, facial cream, or face soap. Use the lotion or soap as you normally would, applying generously to your skin.

For even more added benefits try blending in 1 teaspoon of coconut oil with the mix. Coconut oil is excellent for your skin, and will enhance the benefits you receive from the herbs.

Allow to sit for a few moments, then rinse off. Repeat daily.

Wonder Green

What you will need:

2 teaspoons green tea leaves (dried)

1 teaspoon chamomile leaves (dried)

1 teaspoon dried calendula leaves (dried)

Directions:

Crush the herbs and blend them with either your favorite moisturizing skin lotion, facial cream, or face soap. Use the lotion or soap as you normally would, applying generously to your skin.

For even more added benefits try blending in 1 teaspoon of coconut oil with the mix. Coconut oil is excellent for your skin, and will enhance the benefits you receive from the herbs.

Allow to sit for a few moments, then rinse off. Repeat daily.

Just What You Wanted

What you will need:

1 teaspoon green tea leaves (dried)

1 teaspoon mint leaves (dried)

1 teaspoon calendula leaves (dried)

Directions:

Crush the herbs and blend them with either your favorite moisturizing skin lotion, facial cream, or face soap. Use the lotion or soap as you normally would, applying generously to your skin.

For even more added benefits try blending in 1 teaspoon of coconut oil with the mix. Coconut oil is excellent for your skin, and will enhance the benefits you receive from the herbs.

Allow to sit for a few moments, then rinse off. Repeat daily.

Herbal Paste

What you will need:

2 teaspoons basil leaves (dried)

1 teaspoon parsley leaves (dried)

1 teaspoon dried burdock

Directions:

Crush the herbs and blend them with either your favorite moisturizing skin lotion, facial cream, or face soap. Use the lotion or soap as you normally would, applying generously to your skin.

For even more added benefits try blending in 1 teaspoon of coconut oil with the mix. Coconut oil is excellent for your skin, and will enhance the benefits you receive from the herbs.

Allow to sit for a few moments, then rinse off. Repeat daily.

Sun Spots

What you will need:

2 teaspoons dried dandelion petals (dried)

1 teaspoon lavender petals (dried)

1 teaspoon dried rose petals (dried)

Directions:

Crush the herbs and blend them with either your favorite moisturizing skin lotion, facial cream, or face soap. Use the lotion or soap as you normally would, applying generously to your skin.

For even more added benefits try blending in 1 teaspoon of coconut oil with the mix. Coconut oil is excellent for your skin, and will enhance the benefits you receive from the herbs.

Allow to sit for a few moments, then rinse off. Repeat daily.

Super Saver
What you will need:

1 teaspoon chamomile leaves (dried)

1 teaspoon elder flowers

1 teaspoon eucalyptus leaves (dried)

Directions:

Crush the herbs and blend them with either your favorite moisturizing skin lotion, facial cream, or face soap. Use the lotion or soap as you normally would, applying generously to your skin.

For even more added benefits try blending in 1 teaspoon of coconut oil with the mix. Coconut oil is excellent for your skin, and will enhance the benefits you receive from the herbs.

Allow to sit for a few moments, then rinse off. Repeat daily.

Go Green
What you will need:

2 teaspoons green tea leaves (dried)

1 teaspoon chickweed leaves (dried)

1 teaspoon spearmint leaves (dried)

Directions:

Crush the herbs and blend them with either your favorite moisturizing skin lotion, facial cream, or face soap. Use the lotion or soap as you normally would, applying generously to your skin.

For even more added benefits try blending in 1 teaspoon of coconut oil with the mix. Coconut oil is excellent for your skin, and will enhance the benefits you receive from the herbs.

Allow to sit for a few moments, then rinse off. Repeat daily.

Very Berry Blush
What you will need:

1 teaspoon rose petals (dried)

1 teaspoon crushed cherry pits

1 teaspoon dried raspberry leaves (dried)

Directions:

Crush the herbs and blend them with either your favorite moisturizing skin lotion, facial cream, or face soap. Use the lotion or soap as you normally would, applying generously to your skin.

For even more added benefits try blending in 1 teaspoon of coconut oil with the mix. Coconut oil is excellent for your skin, and will enhance the benefits you receive from the herbs.

Allow to sit for a few moments, then rinse off. Repeat daily.

Skin Toner
What you will need:

1 teaspoon fennel leaves (dried)

2 teaspoons hibiscus leaves (dried)

1 teaspoon dandelion leaves (dried)

Directions:

Crush the herbs and blend them with either your favorite moisturizing skin lotion, facial cream, or face soap. Use the lotion or soap as you normally would, applying generously to your skin.

For even more added benefits try blending in 1 teaspoon of coconut oil with the mix. Coconut oil is excellent for your skin, and will enhance the benefits you receive from the herbs.

Allow to sit for a few moments, then rinse off. Repeat daily.

Toned and Tight
What you will need:

1 teaspoon spearmint leaves (dried)

1 teaspoon chickweed leaves (dried)

1 teaspoon dried rosehips

Directions:

Crush the herbs and blend them with either your favorite moisturizing skin lotion, facial cream, or face soap. Use the lotion or soap as you normally would, applying generously to your skin.

For even more added benefits try blending in 1 teaspoon of coconut oil with the mix. Coconut oil is excellent for your skin, and will enhance the benefits you receive from the herbs.

Allow to sit for a few moments, then rinse off. Repeat daily.

Wrinkle Wonder

What you will need:

1 teaspoon holy basil leaves (dried)

1 teaspoon honeysuckle leaves (dried)

1 teaspoon chamomile leaves (dried)

Directions:

Crush the herbs and blend them with either your favorite moisturizing skin lotion, facial cream, or face soap. Use the lotion or soap as you normally would, applying generously to your skin.

For even more added benefits try blending in 1 teaspoon of coconut oil with the mix. Coconut oil is excellent for your skin, and will enhance the benefits you receive from the herbs.

Allow to sit for a few moments, then rinse off. Repeat daily.

Go for the Gold

What you will need:

1 teaspoon helichrysum leaves (dried)

2 teaspoons goldenrod leaves (dried)

1 teaspoon calendula leaves (dried)

Directions:

Crush the herbs and blend them with either your favorite moisturizing skin lotion, facial cream, or face soap. Use the lotion or soap as you normally would, applying generously to your skin.

For even more added benefits try blending in 1 teaspoon of coconut oil with the mix. Coconut oil is excellent for your skin, and will enhance the benefits you receive from the herbs.

Allow to sit for a few moments, then rinse off. Repeat daily.

Radiant Glow
What you will need:

2 teaspoons lady's mantel leaves (dried)

2 teaspoons juniper berries

Directions:

Crush the herbs and blend them with either your favorite moisturizing skin lotion, facial cream, or face soap. Use the lotion or soap as you normally would, applying generously to your skin.

For even more added benefits try blending in 1 teaspoon of coconut oil with the mix. Coconut oil is excellent for your skin, and will enhance the benefits you receive from the herbs.

Allow to sit for a few moments, then rinse off. Repeat daily.

Cheerfulness

What you will need:

1 teaspoon lavender leaves (dried)

1 teaspoon rose petals (dried)

1 teaspoon lemon balm leaves (dried)

Directions:

Crush the herbs and blend them with either your favorite moisturizing skin lotion, facial cream, or face soap. Use the lotion or soap as you normally would, applying generously to your skin.

For even more added benefits try blending in 1 teaspoon of coconut oil with the mix. Coconut oil is excellent for your skin, and will enhance the benefits you receive from the herbs.

Allow to sit for a few moments, then rinse off. Repeat daily.

Clear Days

What you will need:

2 teaspoons marshmallow leaves (dried)

1 teaspoon licorice leaves (dried)

1 teaspoon neem leaves (dried)

Directions:

Crush the herbs and blend them with either your favorite moisturizing skin lotion, facial cream, or face soap. Use the lotion or soap as you normally would, applying generously to your skin.

For even more added benefits try blending in 1 teaspoon of coconut oil with the mix. Coconut oil is excellent for your skin, and will enhance the benefits you receive from the herbs.

Allow to sit for a few moments, then rinse off. Repeat daily.

Conclusion

There you have it, everything you need to know about herbal and essential oil remedies, and how you can bring it into your skincare regimen on a daily basis. I know you want what's best for your skin, but you also want skin that is youthful, radiant, and blemish free.

You miss the skin you used to have – the skin without the blemishes and wrinkles, the skin without the sun spots and dark circles. You miss the skin that could have been in a skin care commercial – the skin you took for granted without even meaning to.

Now, you have the chance to get that skin back, and this book is going to show you how. There's no end to the ways you can use natural remedies for all your skin care and health care needs. From the remedies that leave you feeling great and ready to take on the world to the remedies that are perfect for sitting back and relaxing, you are going to get what you want with the natural way of life.

Our bodies are designed to use the world around us in ways that synthetic medication could never provide. Though the chemicals seem to give us the results we are looking for, they are actually doing more harm than good, and leaving us with side effects we would rather do without.

I hope this book gives you the inspiration you need to not only turn to herbs and essential oils for your skin care, but for the rest of your needs as well. There's no end to the benefits you are going to experience when you use natural methods to take care of yourself, and the lack of side effects is going to keep you coming back again and again.

The very next time you have an ailment, head to the local health food store and select essential oils and natural remedies, and forget going to the pharmacy where you will spend hours in line for a product that doesn't give you the results you want.

You can now have that skin you miss once more, only this time it's better than ever. You know you work hard, and you don't care for your skin like you should, but all that's about to change. With these recipes, you can pamper yourself like you deserve to be pampered.

So go ahead, indulge in the natural way of life. You deserve a nice break, and that's just what your skin is going to get with these remedies.

Happy pampering.